Cyprus Hearts

Romances for Seniors

seniorality

Cyprus Hearts -
Jamie Stonebridge, Chrissie Stephen

Set in 22 pt EB Garamond

Chapter 1
New Beginnings

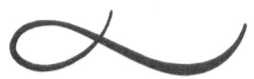

LAURA felt a rush of excitement as she caught her first glimpse of the island of Cyprus through the aircraft window. Far below her, she could see the azure waters of the Mediterranean lapping against small and seemingly deserted golden beaches.

As the pilot adjusted the aircraft's position and started the final descent, Laura could make out the outline of Paphos castle and had a 'bird's eye' view of several little fishing harbors.

The aircraft flew even lower, and within minutes, it had gently landed, eliciting applause from all the Cypriot passengers onboard. Once the aircraft had finished taxiing, the seat belt signs were switched off, the cabin door was swung open and the ground crew gave a cheerful 'welcome to Cyprus' to their passengers.

At nineteen years old, Laura had just quit college in England and found herself at crossroads, not sure in which direction her life would lead. Before college, her life had seemed like an endless adventure made up of different countries and new beginnings.

Her father's long military service had taken them to Germany, Northern

Ireland, Canada, and many different towns England but it had also left her rootless and uncertain of her place in the world.

Because of college in England, Laura had missed out on his latest posting to the Mediterranean island of Cyprus. Today was her first visit.

Laura stood at the top of the aircraft steps and inhaled the fragrance of the island for the first time – it was a distinctive and unforgettable blend of fresh herbs, carried on the warm Mediterranean breeze.

She followed the line of passengers down the aircraft steps and into the terminal to collect her luggage.

Her parents stood by the barrier, eager to spot their eldest daughter. Their reunion was a moment of pure joy, with tight hugs and bright smiles. Suddenly, it felt to Laura that it had been a long time since she had seen them, much longer than just the six months it had been.

Soon they were in the car and her father was driving towards Limassol – a large cosmopolitan town with a reputation for good nightlife. The countryside seemed so different, with sandy-colored soil and scrubby vegetation, and Laura loved its rustic charm.

Laura spotted several shepherds watching their flocks of sheep or goats, with their working dogs lying lazily at their feet. The azure-colored sea was never far away and seemed to stretch to infinity.

After driving for twenty minutes or so, Laura's father turned off the main road and into military housing. The style of houses and the road sign with the words 'Dorset Drive' made them all chuckle - "Oh my goodness, this all looks very English," said Laura.

The houses were all set back from the road with Mediterranean-style front gardens featuring rocky outcrops, huge cacti, and colorful geraniums. They were built in red brick and had pitched red tile roofs.

The effect felt oddly English and familiar but completely out of place amidst the Mediterranean landscape. The houses looked so different from the typical Cypriot houses Laura had seen on the journey that were white-washed and single-story with flat roofs topped by water heaters.

Walking inside, the house felt beautifully cool as her mother had tilted the blinds to keep the sun's rays out. Her mother showed Laura to her bedroom, where she quickly unpacked her clothes. Laura paused and spent time looking out the window, wondering what the coming weeks or even months would bring. She felt she had prepared herself well for her holiday in Cyprus as she had already read about all the popular places to visit, but seeing it for herself filled her with wonder.

Back downstairs, she found her parents sitting outside on the terrace, enjoying some home-made lemonade. Laura sat in a large rattan armchair and spotted a bunch of shiny car keys that had been placed on the table in front of her.

"These are the keys to your mother's car, consider it your holiday rental" said her father, smiling as he pointed to the keys.

"We thought you might enjoy exploring the countryside during your stay to keep yourself busy."

"Driving here is easy as it is just like in England - on the left and with the same style road signs. You'll find many traces of home here as Cyprus used to be a British crown colony," her mother said, encouragingly.

Laura was delighted as she loved to drive and had passed her test as soon as she turned 17 in England. This was a source of endless irritation for her younger sister Katie, who was frustrated that she could not learn to drive in Cyprus until after her 18th birthday in July.

They were so busy talking about Cyprus, the colorful markets, and the beaches that they did not hear footsteps on the garden path that suddenly broke into a run.

"Sis, it's you!"

Katie rushed to warmly embrace her older sister with a huge hug and a shower of exaggerated kisses before also helping herself to a cooling glass of lemonade.

Katie was in her last year at the local British school and was working hard as she was keen to get to university to study law.

Watching her sister pour the lemonade, Laura felt a brief pang of envy as Katie seemed to have her life planned out and because she was bright, she would succeed.

Things hadn't gone quite so well for Laura. She had chosen to take a training course in design. Either the course was not right for her, or she wasn't right for the course because things had not gone well.

It had all become too much a few weeks earlier in a tearful telephone conversation with her parents.

Laura had been surprised at how supportive and understanding her parents had been during that call. They were accepting and acknowledged that sometimes things don't work out how we first think they will.

Her friends had helped her to get her kit packed from college and moved to her Grandma's attic. It was her parents who suggested that she fly over to Cyprus for an extended holiday. Perhaps that the change of scenery would encourage her to find her way.

The next few days passed slowly, and Laura felt herself really beginning to relax. She spent time stretched out on the beach, snoozing in the sunshine and underneath the sun umbrella reading for hours.

Laura tried not to think about the past few months and what had gone wrong as she was sure that the future would present itself when it was ready.

She drove into Limassol town and spent hours browsing the market stalls and taking photographs of the locally grown fruit that glistened in the morning sunshine.

Laura took herself for daily walks along the cliff tops and found herself rediscovering all the simple joys in life.

She had not realized how all-consuming college life had been. How the days had passed without her even noticing the changes in the weather and the arrival of spring.

Her days in England had been filled with boring lectures on the history and different aspects of design, critical thinking, and concept. There was little chance to simply relax in the studio and be creative.

The freedom of having a car and the simple pleasure of driving through the Cypriot countryside and observing was proving therapeutic and energizing. It was helping her to distance herself from the recent upheavals in her life.

Laura decided to drive herself over to the nearby village of Melanda that perched high on a hilltop overlooking the sea. She was looking forward to exploring the village as it was said to be the prettiest in the area, with houses covered in colorful bougainvillea and fragrant honeysuckle.

As Laura traveled, she felt a sense of liberation and wonder at the natural beauty that surrounded her.

Walking through the winding streets of Melanda, Laura was greeted by friendly faces and warm smiles.

She stopped to admire the vibrant colors of the flowers that adorned the houses and the breathtaking views of the sea in the distance.

The village seemed frozen in time, untouched by the hustle and bustle of modern life. Laura found herself enchanted by its charm and restful ambiance.

As she wandered further into the heart of the village, Laura stumbled upon a small coffee shop. The scent of freshly brewed coffee and warm honey-soaked pastries filled the air and was irresistible. She sipped the small cup of coffee, which she found surprisingly strong and understood why it was served with an accompanying glass of water. She savored the warm pastry and then was eager to get back to her exploring.

Laura ventured down some of the side streets and in one, she stumbled across some Cypriot women in a shady courtyard making Halloumi - the local cheese. She watched as they poured a mixture of sheep, goat, and cow's milk into a huge copper cauldron perched above a gas burner.

The oldest woman, a woman in her seventies with silver hair swept into a loose bun, was busy stirring the milk with a huge wooden paddle.

Although they couldn't speak English to Laura and she couldn't speak Greek, they eagerly encouraged her to step forward to watch them work.

Slowly as the liquid heated, Laura could see curds forming, and the woman skillfully stirred the whey so that the curds clumped together. After a few moments, the curds were carefully lifted out with large slotted spoons onto draining racks.

Laura continued to watch the women as they then spooned the soft curds into terracotta pots, carefully pressing down on each cheese to squeeze out any excess whey and to ensure a good shape.

The cheeses were then carefully removed from the pots and dropped back into the cauldron of whey where they were cooked for a further thirty minutes.

During this time, the women were eager to learn about Laura, using mime and the odd word of English to communicate.

They gave her fresh orange juice to drink and a small dish of shiny black olives and there were plenty of smiles and laughter.

Laura felt so welcomed.

When the cooking time was complete, the cheeses were removed from the whey, sprinkled with salt, and garnished with fresh mint.

One piece of cheese was ceremoniously wrapped in grease-proof paper and presented to Laura.

Realizing that it would soon be lunchtime, Laura said goodbye to the women and retraced her steps through the village.

Smelling the wonderful aroma of freshly baked bread in the air, she went in search of the bakery.

The baker was a big burly man dressed in a voluminous white overall with flour dusted on his face. He asked if she would like some bread.

As Laura could only see large circular loaves on display she signaled to him that she would prefer a smaller loaf. In traditional Cypriot style, he dealt with her request in a charming, no-nonsense manner, by reaching for a bread saw and simply cutting a large loaf in two.

Laura was still laughing about this when she put the warm bread and Halloumi into a string bag she found in her mother's car.

She placed the bag on the passenger seat of the car, ready for the next stage of her drive.

Chapter 2
Harvest of the Heart

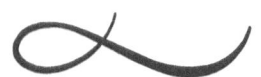

DIMITRI woke to the sound of the rooster crowing, just as he did every morning. He wished he could linger in bed a little longer, but he knew he needed an early start to accomplish as much as possible before the heat of the day set in.

After getting dressed, he went into the kitchen where his mother had prepared a small cup of traditional coffee along with a glass of cool water and a plate of several dry rusks with homemade jam.

Dimitri thanked her and stepped outside onto the terrace to watch the sunrise, his favorite part of the day.

The golden sun was clearly visible above the hills to the east. Dimitri then looked across to the sea in the opposite direction, where he could see numerous small fishing boats bobbing on the waves.

He wondered if his uncle was among the fishermen who would soon be heading for the harbor with their catch.

Taking his plate, cup, and glass back indoors, he bid his mother goodbye and walked through the large sitting room to the front door, where his battered pickup truck was parked just outside.

He drove through the lanes to the outskirts of the village and then along the twisting road that led down to the vineyards and farmland. At the road junction, he turned left and headed inland. Turning right would lead to Melanda Bay with its curved beach of smooth pebbles, the small fishing harbor, and the rustic bars and taverns he liked to visit.

He crossed the old main road and gazed at the family's vineyards ahead. Not for the first time, he felt a swell of pride as he thought of his grandfather, who had spent his so much time planting all the vines by hand many years before.

Driving along, he reflected on his grandfather's name – Dimitri – and the local tradition of naming the firstborn son after the grandfather. His parents had followed this tradition when he was born.

Dimitri chuckled at the thought of the name's appropriateness, originating from Demeter – the ancient Greek goddess of the harvest.

Dimitri stopped the truck and unlocked the padlock on the gates before getting back into the driver's seat to maneuver the truck into the shade of the vine canopy in front of their small workroom.

It was time to start work; the air was already losing its morning coolness.

There was plenty to be done before his father, Petros, arrived to inspect the vines in the mid-afternoon. Petros would already be at work in the winery, which was a few kilometers further along the main road.

Dimitri smiled as he thought of his father carefully inspecting the wine vats, nurturing the different wines as though they were his babies.

Dimitri grabbed his hand tools and then walked to the first row of vines. They were growing rapidly now.

He remembered how strenuous the earlier pruning work had been. Dimitri and his father had worked long hours together to get it done, sustained by abundant food carefully packed by their mother.

Pruning was time-consuming but essential to keep the vines strong. If left unchecked, the vines would produce too many bunches of grapes, resulting in lower quality fruit.

The pruning had been completed during the final weeks of winter when there was still snow on the Troodos Mountain tops.

They had been relieved to finish the work then, as unexpectedly mild weather had suddenly arrived, pushing away the winter and bringing early spring.

Dimitri walked slowly through the vines, meticulously checking that they were all properly supported and that the new growth was thriving. In a couple of places, he added long green ties to secure the leafy shoots firmly in place.

With over a thousand vines to tend to, this occupied much of Dimitri's morning.

He was eager to also check the condition of the soil before taking a well-deserved lunch break.

It was crucial to regularly test the soil and adjust the pH levels to optimize the nutrients provided to the vines.

Dimitri noticed that after the light rains the previous week, he would have plenty of weed growth to cut back. He knew he wouldn't have time to look at this later when his father arrived, as they needed to discuss the plans for the summer irrigation system.

More quickly than he would have liked, Dimitri heard the church bells from Melanda village strike twelve and knew he must work quickly to test the soil. As he walked to the workshop, he felt beads of perspiration forming on his forehead and wondered how high the summer temperatures would rise.

He retrieved a pot and trowel from the workshop and headed over to the first row of vines. Carefully, he dug a small hole the length of his hand and collected a few teaspoons of soil.

Back in the workroom, he carefully placed the soil in a clear glass jar and poured in some distilled water. He firmly screwed the metal top on the jar and shook it vigorously. Then, he carefully undid the lid and drained the water from the soil.

He reached for a pH test strip from the shelf and was pleased when he saw the reading was well within the acceptable range. He announced loudly to himself that he had definitely earned his lunch and whistled as he locked the door and gate behind him.

Dimitri always looked forward to his lunch break. He would take the packed lunch his mother had prepared for him, lock up the vineyard and stroll along the main road to the far end of the vines.

Behind a small dirt car park, there was a large open area used for animal grazing. Dimitri enjoyed nothing more than walking along the earth path to a jumbled circle of stones under a huge carob tree on the far side. It was the perfect spot to stretch out in the shade and unwind.

He often found that he shared his lunch spot with the local shepherd. His family had known Savvas for years and Dimitri enjoyed the lively political debates he had with the older man. The two men would place all their food packages on the shaded grass between them so they could share their meal. Dimitri was always very happy to do this, as Savvas usually had a chunk of good lounza smoked ham in his lunch.

Dimitri arrived at the shepherd's rest, and a flash of disappointment crossed his brow when he saw that he was alone.

He folded his sweatshirt to make a cushion for himself, then quickly unpacked his lunch, as his stomach growled with hunger.

His mother certainly knew how to prepare a feast fit for a king, as she had cut thick slices of village bread to dip in the pot of creamy homemade hummus made with chickpeas.

In another package, there were slices of cold sausage, and in a small brown paper bag, the season's new apricots with their soft, smooth skins.

Once he finished his meal, Dimitri swiftly repacked the food to protect it from any ants.

Although tempted to stretch out and rest, he was mindful of the local folklore. It was said that while sleeping under an olive tree was good for dreams, anyone who dared to sleep under a carob tree would not enjoy a peaceful rest.

34

Chapter 3
A Chance Meeting

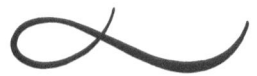

IN KEEPING with his usual routine, Dimitri unfolded a copy of yesterday's newspaper that his father had left for him on the kitchen table this morning. Glancing at his watch, he began to study the sports pages.

To him, this was the ideal break after lunchtime, especially as the thick, dark leaves of the carob tree shaded him perfectly from the sun.

After a while, he became aware that someone was walking towards him, a young lady with long brown hair and a slim figure.

Her skin was very pale - the color of porcelain - which surprised him. She certainly didn't look tanned or local.

As she approached the edge of the stones, he smiled and said "Kalimera," meaning "Good afternoon" in Greek.

Laura had been lost in her own thoughts and had not spotted Dimitri sitting among the stones, especially as his green work pants and cream tee shirt blended into the surroundings so well.

When he spoke, she jumped, but quickly repeated, "Kalimera," and gave him a shy smile.

"Are you English?" Dimitri asked curiously.

"I am," said Laura. "Do you speak English?"

Dimitri laughed and said he tries to.

He explained that all schoolchildren learn English at school in Cyprus, and he enjoyed reading English books but that rarely had the chance to practice his English.

He also mentioned that he listened to pop music on the British Forces radio station, BFBS, where he heard English DJs introduce the songs and read the news.

"Why have you stopped here?" he asked. "Where are you going?"

Laura explained that she had been visiting the village of Melanda. She described her morning with the women making Halloumi and then her visit to the bakery to buy some bread.

She ended her summary by saying, "I remembered seeing the parking place when I drove to the village and thought it would be fun to explore and find somewhere to enjoy my lunch."

Dimitri got up to introduce himself and offered Laura his folded sweatshirt to sit on.

He stretched out his hand, and Laura took it. As she shook his hand, she was surprised by how strong and firm his handshake was.

"Thank you, Dimitri. Would you like to share some of the fresh bread and Halloumi?" she offered.

Dimitri told her that he would and started laughing as he explained that he lived in the village of Melanda and had realized that the Halloumi makers had probably included his own mother and her sister.

Laura opened the two packages she had been carrying in the string bag. Dimitri took his pen knife from his bag, wiped the blade and expertly cut several slices of Halloumi and two thick pieces of bread.

They ate the food in a relaxed silence before Dimitri asked Laura his first question, "Do you live in Cyprus, Lowra?" as he struggled to say her name.

Laura explained that she was on an extended holiday and staying with her parents, quite close by, near a small village called Paramali.

She giggled and tried to explain to Dimitri as gently as possible the correct pronunciation of her name – little knowing that it would prove a real challenge for him to get right.

In the shade of the carob tree, Dimitri proudly told Laura about the family's vineyards and how his grandfather had first planted all the vines and built the small winery further along the main road.

He described how his grandfather was now taking life at a leisurely pace and preferred to walk each day to the coffee shop in the village square to meet with his friends to discuss the day's politics.

Dimitri explained how he and his father now ran the business together.

His grandfather had run the vineyard and winery for years but had announced that as soon as his grandson Dimitri had completed his military service, it would be the ideal time for him to take life a little easier.

Dimitri had totally agreed with the idea and had started work just before his twenty-first birthday. He was now twenty-three years old and took pride in his work.

He expressed his hopes and dreams for the future too, which included going abroad to study winemaking and building a larger winery.

Dimitri reflected on how the wine business in Cyprus was rapidly changing.

In the early days, most of the winemakers grew local grape varieties and used traditional winemaking methods. Today, Dimitri explained, there were several winemakers who had made huge investments, importing the latest winemaking equipment from all over Europe, including large stainless-steel vats from Germany.

Certainly, winemaking had changed dramatically and had become a true science.

Dimitri laughed when Laura asked him whether the standard of Cyprus wines had improved because of these changes in the industry. He explained how the new wines were excellent, especially as new grape varieties were now being grown and blended with the indigenous varieties with great success.

Laura was enchanted by this talkative, friendly man. She found it all so fascinating and there was plenty of laughter as she gently helped him with his English pronunciation.

In mid-sentence Dimitri suddenly looked at his watch and gasped. How time had flown! Standing up, he apologized, but would have to leave her and get back to work as his father would be arriving at the vineyard soon and there was still much to be done.

Feeling guilty about being so abrupt, he helped Laura to her feet, before picking up his sweatshirt and passing her the string bag. He walked her to her car, repeating his apologies whilst wishing he could have stayed with her for longer. It seemed they both felt a kind of connection.

Once at the car, Laura opened the door, and they paused, both looking at each other for a moment before quickly saying goodbye.

As Laura climbed into the car, Dimitri took a chance and asked her if she was free the following day and whether she would like to meet in the same place for lunch at one p.m. Laura blushed and said that she certainly would really like that.

As Laura drove out of the parking area, she spotted a winery lorry heading in the opposite direction and smiled to herself at the thought of Dimitri rushing around getting everything ready for his father.

She continued her drive towards her parents' house and realized that she was thinking only of Dimitri and reliving the past hour – it had made her feel so alive.

As she looked in her rearview mirror, she noticed for the first time that her cheeks were a little red and flushed.

An hour or so later, her mother's footsteps could be heard on the garden path. Laura was sitting in the leafy shade of the terrace, daydreaming whilst trying to read a book.

Her mother smiled and went inside, returning with a tray holding a jug of lemonade and two glasses. She sat opposite Laura and as she handed her a glass of chilled lemonade.

"Did you enjoy your trip to Melanda?" she asked.

"Yes, it was fascinating, very rustic. I had no idea there were so many places growing vines. I might go back tomorrow with my camera to take some photographs," Laura replied.

Much as she wanted to tell her mother about Dimitri, Laura felt it best not to.

She suspected that her recent experience of dropping out of college had disappointed her parents, even if they had said otherwise.

She thought it best to keep sharing an impromptu lunch with Dimitri to herself, for now at least.

Anyway, she had only met him by accident, and yet she did admit to herself that he was very charming and couldn't wait to see what tomorrow might bring.

Chapter 4
Sips of Romance

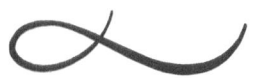

LAURA was not surprised that she woke up early the next morning. She knew herself well enough to know that the minutes would drag their feet.

She decided that she should fill her morning by doing something constructive, and what better idea than to visit the wine museum in Erimi as 'homework'.

Laura had carefully written down the opening hours and directions in her notebook. Checking with her mother about the journey time, she decided that it would be best to drive straight from the museum to the vineyard afterwards. She also packed her camera.

Laura asked her mother if she could use the cool box and carefully removed the remaining Halloumi and some bottles of cold water from the fridge, popping them into the cool box with some ice blocks.

She said goodbye to her mother, who was leaving for work in the Army's newspaper office.

Soon, Laura was on her way. She decided to take the old road rather than the highway as she wanted to see how the road followed the coastline.

The road carved its way through scrubby heathland, and she stopped to take photographs of golden-flowered gorse, myrtle, rosemary, and Aleppo pines. The road led past the Army base to a small village.

Laura parked next to the grocery store. She had visited it a few days earlier with her mother and thought it was the ideal place to pick up some food for lunch.

Outside the store front were numerous wooden boxes piled high with glistening fresh fruit and vegetables.

When Laura stepped inside the store, she certainly stepped back in time. The floor was dry earth, and all the products were stacked on old wooden shelves in a haphazard way.

The store was lit by sunlight that found its way through gaps in the roof. Yiannis, the proprietor, was quite a fun character who liked to laugh, joke, and practice his English.

Amazingly, he knew where every single product was stored.

The first time Laura had seen the array of fresh produce with her mother, she had laughed when she spotted that it was all sold with leaves still attached. She had chosen some large, juicy oranges – each with a stalk and two dark shiny leaves.

Today she took a small brown paper bag and filled it with beautiful dark red cherries that Yiannis explained were the first of the year and had been brought to his shop fresh from the mountains.

Laura added some warm pitta bread, large tomatoes, and small Cyprus-style cucumbers to her shopping basket. She also bought some kourambiedes - delicious almond shortbreads dusted with icing sugar.

Once back at the car, she safely stored the food she had bought into the cool box. She drove away from the shop, amused at the contrast between it and all the large, brightly lit stores she knew in England.

Shortly, Laura arrived at the Erimi Wine Museum. It looked impressive as it was in a large and elegant mellow colored stone building that stood overlooking a wide dry river valley – just as it had done for several centuries.

Laura gasped with surprise when she stepped into the museum as it was very impressive with excellent displays and photographs bathed in a golden light.

As she walked into the first room, a lady was walking towards her. She introduced herself as Maria.

Maria spoke good English, and as the museum was quiet, she gave Laura a private tour.

She explained that the island of Cyprus had been linked with wine production for more than 5,000 years, and it was the first place in Europe where wine was produced.

She pointed to a large map on the wall that showed where the wine museum stands today, marking the very first place where wines were produced in Europe – a fact that had been verified by archaeologists who examined an ancient stone storage wine jar found locally.

Laura thoroughly enjoyed her time at the museum, which included outside in the courtyard. She also learned it was sometimes the setting for musical performances and special events during the summer months.

The tour ended at a wine gift shop, and Laura bought a bottle of red wine for her father. The thought crossed her mind that she must ask Dimitri for the name of his winery.

After she had enjoyed the wine museum, Laura was back in the car heading for Melanda.

She decided to take the highway for the return journey to ensure she reached the vineyard in good time to meet Dimitri.

As she approached the turning, she looked across and could see the village high on its hilltop, with the beautiful Mediterranean beyond.

Laura parked the car in the parking area and carried the cool box to the circle of stones under the carob trees. She ran back to the car to collect the tartan rug from the back seat and her camera.

Once back at the stones, she worked quickly to make the picnic area look welcoming.

She sat down and took her book out of her bag to read, but realized that while she was reading the words, her brain was not absorbing any of them. About ten minutes later, she heard footsteps and Dimitri's voice calling, "Kalimera – good afternoon."

She stood up and walked towards him, and they gently shook hands, although this time their hands remained clasped for a few extra moments.

They sat down in the leafy shade of the tree. Laura carefully placed the various bags of food on the tartan rug, and Dimitri supplemented the array with several pots of homemade dips that his mother had made early that morning.

Over their picnic, Laura and Dimitri talked about their mornings.

Dimitri had spent his time weeding around each vine and checking the leaves for signs of any pests, as these could ruin a vineyard in no time at all.

Laura told Dimitri about her visit to the wine museum. Dimitri was impressed with what she told him and had many questions as it was a place that he had not yet visited. At this point, Laura teased him as she asked him why not, as it had clearly been there for many years.

Once they had finished their lunch, Dimitri asked her to close her eyes, explaining that he had learned in his lessons at school that this is how you gave an English person a surprise.

Laura closed her eyes, but after a few moments asked if she could open them, to which Dimitri replied, "Not yet."

Eventually, Dimitri invited her to open her eyes, and on a small silver tray stood two small pretty glasses that were half-filled with red wine.

"I know you are driving later, but I wanted to share our first small glass of wine together," Dimitri explained.

He handed her a glass and then took one for himself. He raised his glass in the air and moved it towards Laura as he said the toast, "Is-iyia - Cheers."

Laura sipped the wine – it tasted wonderful. It was vibrant and delicate at the same time, it tasted all the more special to be drinking it on the land where the grapes had been grown, and in the company of Dimitri.

They continued to talk about the wine museum and all that Laura had seen.

Eventually Dimitri plucked up the courage to ask, "Laura, I would really like to take you out to dinner tomorrow evening. Please will you come? There is a fish restaurant overlooking the beach and sea, just a few kilometers from here.

It is a very special place, and I think you will like it very much."

Laura searched her thoughts and quickly agreed that she would really enjoy dinner by the sea and the chance to spend more time with him.

Dimitri explained to her that dinner in Cyprus was later than in other countries and asked if 8 p.m. would suit her as it would give him the chance to finish work and change his clothes.

They agreed to meet by the small fishing harbor, and Dimitri explained to her how easy it was to drive there.

It was now time for Dimitri to return to work. They carefully packed away the picnic, and Dimitri wrapped the empty glasses carefully in towels, placing them in his bag.

They walked slowly back to Laura's car, Dimitri carrying the folded tartan rug. As they put everything in the trunk, Dimitri asked if she had time to see the vineyard.

Together they walked on the grass at the side of the road, and Dimitri opened the padlock on the gate. He showed her the rows of vines and Laura took some photographs of the landscape before he walked her back to the car.

They said goodbye awkwardly, neither wanting the moment to end. Dimitri wished her a happy afternoon, reminding her about their plans for the following evening.

Laura stood and watched him as he walked back along the side of the road towards the vineyard.

Once in the car, she decided not to break the spell and drive home but to experience a little more of Cyprus.

She drove along to the harbor that Dimitri had described instead.

Laura was enchanted with what she saw. The harbor was small, with a dozen brightly painted fishing boats bobbing by the wooden jetty. She took photographs of the beach, with its smooth, rounded pebbles that stretched on either side of the jetty, forming a large arc.

Turning around and gazing inland, Laura could see Melanda village on the hilltop and endless vineyards in the valley.

She returned to the car with her mind filled with thoughts about Dimitri, the wine museum and dreaming of their dinner date the following night.

That evening, when she sat at the table with her parents and her sister Katie, she described her day in full.

She gave her father the bottle of wine she had bought and explained why she had chosen to go to the wine museum. She told them about meeting Dimitri, how friendly he was, and about his invitation to dinner.

Her family seemed very happy for her, as if they could sense that the difficulties she had experienced at college were now in the past. Laura seemed to glow with growing confidence and happiness.

Chapter 5
Cyprus Embrace

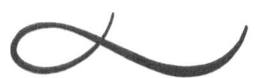

THE FOLLOWING evening, when Laura drove into the harbor car park, she saw that Dimitri was already there and in deep conversation with a fisherman.

Laura walked shyly towards them, and Dimitri took her by the arm, guiding her towards the older man, proudly introducing him as his uncle.

The men carried on talking for a few moments before, with a warm wave, the fisherman walked along the wooden jetty and jumped down onto his fishing boat.

Dimitri held Laura's arm to guide her towards the furthest tavern. Dimitri pointed to a table right by the beach, declaring that he had chosen the "ring top" table just for Laura. She laughed and gently corrected his English, saying that he meant the "ringside table" because it was closest to the sea and all the activity in the harbor.

From their table they could see Dimitri's uncle heading out to sea, and there seemed to be dozens of assorted boats following him.

They were still watching when the waiter came to the table with the menus, which were written in Greek.

Dimitri tried his best to describe each of the dishes in turn, and not for the first time, he reprimanded himself for not having made more of an effort in his English classes.

Laura felt very comfortable in Dimitri's company, and the meal passed easily as they found so much to talk about.

The waiter brought a carafe of red wine to the table and poured two glasses. Dimitri watched intently as Laura took her first sips and laughed when she told him that the wine was very similar to the one they had yesterday.

Dimitri proudly told her that it was the same wine and that all the taverns by the harbor stocked their three wines – two reds and a new rosé.

They ate warm bread that was served with olive oil as a starter, followed by a local feta cheese salad, stuffed vine leaves and the freshest grilled fish Laura had ever eaten.

With the gentle rhythms of the harbor and the warm evening air, it was such a relaxing experience that time just flew by.

At the end of the meal, the waiter brought some chilled peaches to the table, announcing that they were the first of the season. He also gave them two small cups of strong coffee and glasses of water. It was a charming end to a delightful meal.

Afterwards they strolled along the wooden jetty and stood gazing out to sea, looking at the lanterns that lit up the fishing boats in the moonlight.

Dimitri slipped his hand into Laura's, and it felt strong, warm, and comforting.

As they slowly walked towards the car park, he gently pulled Laura towards him, wrapped his arms around her, and they kissed.

It was a moment that made them both feel like time stood still, that they were the only two people in the whole island of Cyprus that mattered.

Over the next few weeks, Laura and Dimitri met regularly for picnic lunches among the shepherd's stones and evening strolls along the harbor or meals in the local taverns.

On weekends, the couple spent their time exploring Cyprus together. They admired Roman mosaics and stood enthralled on the huge stone stage of a Roman theater perched high on the sea cliffs.

They visited numerous wine villages, the mountains, and swam at sandy beaches.

Laura's parents were delighted that their elder daughter seemed so relaxed and happy.

One evening, they raised the subject of Laura's plans for the future and when she would be returning to England.

Laura admitted that these were questions she had put out of her mind and decisions she knew she should have to make.

Over the next week or so, Laura spent a great deal of time thinking things through but didn't come to any conclusion. Her relationship with Dimitri felt very special, but it was still in its beginnings, and she felt it was too soon to be planning a future together.

A few days later, they were enjoying a picnic on a huge sandy beach called Coral Bay. It was certainly a popular beach, and there were numerous holidaymakers enjoying the warm evening.

Dimitri had mentioned to Laura that he had chosen to take her to Coral Bay because the sunsets on the western side of the island were particularly spectacular, and he was not wrong.

The large golden orb of the sun began to sink slowly in the sky in the early evening, turning the thin strips of wispy clouds a rich and shimmering color.

Like others on the beach, Laura and Dimitri sat together and simply watched as the sun slowly sank beyond the horizon. As there is no dusk in Cyprus, once the sun goes down, the night immediately arrives with its inky blackness.

After they had sat, with Laura's head resting on Dimitri's shoulder, they walked over to one of the beach bars and ordered drinks.

When the drinks had arrived at their table, Dimitri turned serious and asked Laura about her plans and whether she had decided when she would be returning to England.

He quickly explained in a jumble of emotional words that he was not suggesting she leave, and that he didn't want her to go because he would miss her far too much.

Suddenly, he leaned across the table and took her hand in his. "S'agapó, Laura. I love you," he said.

They found that his declaration of love gave them both new confidence, and they started to talk freely about the future.

Dimitri explained he had long dreamed of going to Athens to study oenology so he could take the family wine business to the next stage.

Laura would return to England. She wondered if it would be good for her to study how to teach English as a second language and take a course in conversational Greek – thereby providing her with the means to no longer be just a tourist.

They had so much to talk about and plans to make.

The next few days and weeks were spent researching the various possibilities and seeing if they could turn their ideas into reality.

They wanted to ensure that if they both started studying, they could return to Cyprus as often as possible to see each other. But top of the list of priorities was for Laura's parents to meet Dimitri.

Laura discussed their ideas with her parents, who were both cautiously encouraging about how both Cyprus and Dimitri had captured her heart.

Laura's mother commented that it would be wonderful to invite Dimitri over for dinner to meet him properly, while her father joked about his delight at him being a winemaker.

In Dimitri's home, similar discussions took place. While his parents seemed pleased about his ideas to grow the wine business and his relationship with Laura, they were also concerned that she was unfamiliar with Greek-Cypriot culture and could not speak the Greek language.

The best news for Laura and Dimitri was that their studies did not start until September, so they had the summer ahead of them to deepen their love.

Laura had found suitable courses for both teaching English and learning Greek close to where her Grandma lived in England.

She telephoned her to ask if she could live with her for a year, and her Grandma could hardly contain her excitement – she was so overjoyed.

Her grandmother also found her a part-time job in the local flower shop so Laura could earn extra money for all the air tickets to Cyprus she would be buying.

That first summer, the days seemed endless and were filled with fun and happiness.

Laura and Dimitri spent time at each other's homes, getting to know each other's parents and family traditions. Neither of them had realized that there were so many subtle cultural differences to learn.

The second time she had visited Dimitri's parents, Laura felt welcome enough to carry the dirty plates from the dining table to the kitchen and to start to wash the dishes.

She suddenly felt eyes watching her and spun around to find Dimitri's family staring at her with their mouths open in surprise.

Dimitri stood next to them laughing. It turned out that in Cyprus, guests never help clear the dinner table and never do the dishes.

They also explained that a large bowl of soapy water is never used, as water is a such a precious commodity on the island, and as little as possible was used for cleaning.

Like the first summer for all young lovers, before they knew it, September had arrived.

Dimitri volunteered to take Laura to the airport, as he would be leaving for

Athens a couple of days later. They knew it was going to be incredibly difficult to be apart - especially the first few weeks as they adjusted to the distance.

They had both booked their first flights back to Cyprus for one month later to make things easier. As Laura's father commented, "Thank heavens for economy airlines."

At the check-in, everything went smoothly and all too quickly. Laura found herself standing at the entrance marked 'Departures and Security.'

She turned to Dimitri, who put his arms around her so tightly that she almost couldn't breathe.

He whispered how much he loved her, and she whispered the same. They promised to send each other messages every day and to call as often as possible.

Unknown to Laura, Dimitri didn't drive away from the airport straight away. Instead, he walked along the perimeter fence to a good spot overlooking the runway.

He watched the passengers climb the steps to the aircraft and thought he recognized Laura in her pretty pink top.

He was so absorbed in his thoughts that he did not notice the aircraft start to move, and it took him by surprise.

As he watched the wheels of the aircraft leave the ground, he felt tears forming in his eyes. He steadied his heart and reminded himself of the great future they had planned.

Chapter 6
Trials of Love

THE TIME apart certainly proved to be a challenge for both Laura and Dimitri.

There were some unbearable moments when they simply missed each other so much they thought they would burst, yet as the days passed, they adapted.

The best part of each day was the telephone call they shared just before bedtime.

Laura quickly settled into her new routine and was grateful to have her grandmother there for company.

She filled her days with study, jumping on and off buses, and working in the flower shop.

There were still plenty of moments when a smell or sound would set her mind wandering to Cyprus.

She found she easily took to the course on teaching English as a second language and she felt she had a natural ability as an instructor.

During the coffee breaks between lessons, she discovered that all the students had one thing in common – they were moving to a country where they didn't know the language. For all of them, teaching English would be the ideal first job.

Laura found her evening classes in Greek much more difficult. She had enrolled in an evening course at the nearest university, but after a few weeks, she felt lost in a sea of seemingly impossible grammar rules.

She began to feel increasingly frustrated because she was trying so hard, but still felt incapable of really speaking the language.

It did not help that Aria, her teacher, was from mainland Greece. She explained that the Greek-Cypriot dialect was quite different, and there were often completely different words for the same thing.

Aria would often say a sentence to the class and then add, "and this is how you would say it in Cyprus," repeating the phrase differently.

To Laura, it felt like she had to learn everything twice, but nevertheless, she persevered. She knew it was essential to be able to speak Greek for the future she and Dimitri had planned.

Dimitri found his course equally demanding but he thrived on it. He appreciated that it was essential for him to learn about all the new ideas and technology, as the result would be better wines that were consistently good. He well remembered that in the past, the same wine could vary greatly from one year to the next – and this wasn't caused just by the weather.

He enjoyed speaking with the other students to learn their approaches to making wine and discuss what they had been taught in their lectures.

Dimitri put all his efforts into studying because he felt that his whole family's future depended on the success of the winery. He also wanted to show Laura that he would be the perfect husband she deserved.

Meeting as often as they could in Cyprus for long weekends certainly was their lifeline. They both sensed their increasing excitement as the day of their flights approached.

As the flight times were usually very different, Laura's father would meet her at the airport. Each time the flight crew opened the cabin door, Laura was delighted to smell the fragrance of wild herbs in the air once again.

The time they had together seemed to race by, but it was always enjoyable.

They found that the time they spent apart made them closer when they were together.

Dimitri had a large family, so there were several weddings and baptisms to attend.

He always proudly introduced Laura to his relatives. They were always curious that she was English, but were delighted when she bravely attempted to speak to them in Greek.

Laura seemed to charm all of them with her affection for Dimitri and her love for Cyprus.

For the first wedding she attended, she had carefully carried a beautiful blue hat with feathers all the way from England in her hand luggage.

When Dimitri came to collect her from her parents' home, he beamed with pride at how lovely she looked, but then started to giggle.

"Your hat is very pretty and also very English, but we don't wear hats at weddings in Cyprus!" he said.

He insisted all the same that she wore it, as he wanted everyone to know how special and different she was. To him, she was his English princess.

While the days they had together were fun, saying 'goodbye' each time became harder.

Luckily, over Christmas and Easter, they were able to stay a few more days in Cyprus together.

Dimitri thoroughly enjoyed learning all the British Christmas traditions and found setting the Christmas pudding on fire with flaming brandy to be unforgettable.

In turn, Laura learned that Cypriots did not really celebrate Christmas, but instead, New Year was the holiday they celebrated as the feast day of Saint Basil.

That New Year's Eve, Dimitri took Laura and her family down to Melanda Bay to watch the firework display, and afterwards they returned to Dimitri's home to share wine and the New Year's cake with his family.

To his surprise and delight, Laura's father found the hidden lucky coin in his slice of traditional cake. He was congratulated by everyone, as finding the coin assured him of good luck for the forthcoming year – something he was sure would include Laura's happiness.

A few months later, Laura and her family were swept into the Easter celebrations.

They went to the midnight mass in Melanda, and the next day, joined in the largest barbecue imaginable, with the entire village cooking whole lambs on spits over pits of glowing charcoal.

Afterwards, everyone relaxed in the April sunshine before the games and dancing began.

On the drive home, Laura's father proclaimed it to have been the best Easter ever, and Katie added that she would not be able to eat for a week as there had been so much food.

It was heartening to see both families, English and Greek, having so much fun and being so comfortable together.

By June, Laura and Dimitri were both back in Cyprus as they had successfully completed their studies and their separation was over.

On their first weekend together, Dimitri gave her flowers, and they went for dinner at their favorite tavern by the harbor in Melanda.

It was a perfect evening; it felt as if they were actors starring in a play made just for the two of them.

In the silver moonlight, Dimitri asked Laura to marry him.

The next few months were an exciting blur of wedding preparations.

Laura spent time with the village priest who prepared her for baptism into the Greek Orthodox Church so they could marry in the traditional way.

As they would be having a Cypriot wedding, Dimitri's parents were happy to organize much of it, but Laura's parents were also involved so they could bring a little bit of English style to the Mediterranean.

Laura, her younger sister Katie, and their mother went shopping in Limassol for a wedding dress.

Katie was to be the chief bridesmaid and was brimming with pride. They spent the whole day trying on a variety of different outfits until they found the one that was just right.

Laura made sure that the bridesmaid dresses were available in smaller sizes too, as there were several flower girls in Dimitri's family.

The wedding day itself was perfect with deep blue skies, warm sunshine, and the beautiful jacaranda trees in bloom.

Laura felt as if she was in a dream, a dream full of love and acceptance.

The church in Melanda was packed to overflowing because Dimitri's family was well known in the village.

Many of Laura's relatives had flown over from England for the occasion, including her Grandma, who had been so supportive during Laura's studies in England.

The wedding service felt truly magical, and Dimitri, her 'prince', looked so handsome.

Laura looked at him often during the service, especially when his Koumbaros or Best Man was placing the floral wedding crowns on their heads three times. The crowns were joined by a ribbon to signify their union as man and wife.

Out in the sunshine, they were showered in fragrant rose petals before they walked together to the village square which had been filled with tables ready for the party to begin.

The wine from the family winery certainly flowed freely that night, as the whole village celebrated the marriage of Laura and Dimitri.

After they had honeymooned in the mountains, Dimitri took Laura by the hand and led her to their new home.

Laura let out a squeal of delight when she saw it was the house with the big shady yard where she had watched the women making Halloumi cheese when she had first come to Cyprus.

The walls of their new home had all been freshly whitewashed, and the wooden shutters had been given a coat of sky-blue paint. It was perfect.

On their front door, two horseshoes had been nailed – one facing up, the other facing down. Dimitri explained the reason why.

"Your father said to me that he found it strange that all the horseshoes he saw in

Cyprus were nailed upside down, so all the good luck pours out," he said.

"I explained to him that because the Cypriots are generous, we nail them upside down so that good luck is sprinkled on everyone. I nailed the second horseshoe the English way so that we keep plenty of good luck for ourselves, always."

Epilogue

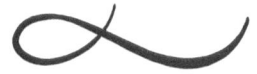

IN THE YEARS that followed, Dimitri expanded the winery buildings and installed state-of-the-art wine-making equipment that still kept true to the traditions passed down through the generations.

His father took on a junior role in the business as Dimitri found new customers and received awards for the quality of their wine.

With the help of their friends from the village, they built a beautiful visitors center with mellow stone walls.

During the tourist season, Laura worked in the visitors center and regularly welcomed coaches of tourists who were eager to learn about the history of Cypriot wine – just as she had been a few years earlier.

To add to their fun and enjoyment, Laura would serve them all with a small glass of red wine for them to taste.

At other times, Laura could be found sitting in the leafy shade of the courtyard of their home, giving English lessons to schoolchildren.

She spent time with her mother-in-law too, learning how to cook all the delicious Cypriot dishes that Dimitri loved so much. On other occasions, she would bake an English cake for the family to enjoy- which they all loved.

The years passed, and Dimitri and Laura had two little boys of their own, each proudly baptized with the name of their grandfathers – Andreas and Richard.

They were happy children who were totally bilingual and able to speak Greek and English fluently.

The children spent much time with their Cypriot grandmother, as Laura's parents by this time had returned to England. However, the family would spend the Christmas holidays in England, enjoying time with their

English family and even the colder, wintry weather.

The boys spent hours in the vineyards with their father, learning the basics about winemaking from an early age so that they could continue the family tradition.

They enjoyed visiting the winery too, where their grandfather proudly showed them all the huge wine-filled vats and the rows of oak barrels in the cellar. He also showed his grandsons all the neatly written ledgers that he now kept, describing to them how much winemaking had changed since he was a boy and how life was all about change and growth.

Life was full and happy for the busy young family.

Often when the children were sleeping at their grandparents' house, Dimitri would prepare a picnic and take Laura to the circle of stones where they had first met.

He would pour two glasses of wine, just as he had done on that first occasion.

He would hand Laura one glass, while he raised the other and said "Is-iyia, yamas agapi-mou - cheers, my love, here's to our wonderful life..."

The End

www.ingramcontent.com/pod-product-compliance
Lightning Source LLC
Chambersburg PA
CBHW050402290526
45786CB00003B/1088